CW00400575

Get My Curls Back!

HOW TO TRANSITION FROM DAMAGED TO HEALTHY NATURAL CURLY HAIR

By Shannon Fitzsimmons

© 2017 Shannon Fitzsimmons. All rights reserved.

Visit the authors website at www. Ukcurlygirl . com

Front Cover Photography by Jade Keshia Gordon @ JKG Photography

Front Cover Makeup by Georgia Mshults @ georg . mshults

All rights reserved. No part of this book may be reproduced in any form or by any means including electronic, mechanical or photocopying or stored in a retrieval system without permission in writing from the publisher except by a reviewer who may quote brief passages to be included in a review.

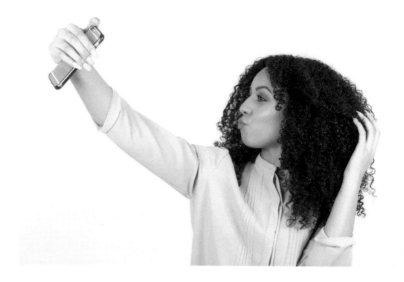

Shannon Fitzsimmons 'UK Curly Girl' is a blogger of mixed race origin born in London, UK.

She shares her knowledge of natural curly hair with girls all around the world via the internet.

In 2013 she created her blog and has now reached over 20,000 followers across all platforms along with working with brands and fellow influencers within the natural hair community.

Her mission is to inspire women to love their natural selves in a world that celebrates perfection.

CHAPTERS

CURLY HAIR DICTIONARY

Before we get started let me fill you in on some of the words and phrases that may be mentioned throughout this book and during your own hair journey.

No Poo – Cutting out shampoo/A cleansing product that is not shampoo.

Low Poo – A mild shampoo.

Wash And Go – Washing your hair and styling it with your curls out in their natural state (The go means you are all washed and ready to step out the door!).

Finger Curls – The method of creating perfect curls by twirling the hair around your finger with a styling product, once dried you have ringlets that you can separate for volume.

Air Dry – Letting your hair dry naturally without a towel or hairdryer.

Rake – Forming your fingers like a rake and applying hair products through the hair this way.

LOC/LCO Method – L=Liquid O=Oil C=Cream. This is a 3 step process of applying products for maximum moisture.

ACV - Apple Cider Vinegar.

JBCO - Jamaican Black Castor Oil.

Co-Wash – Washing your hair with conditioner.

Big Chop – Cutting off all of your damaged/relaxed hair.

Elasticity – The measure of how much your curls will stretch and then pop back to its   normal state. Healthy hair will have great elasticity.

Porosity – The hairs ability to absorb moisture.

Curl Envy – The feeling of wanting someone else's curls more than your own.

1
INTRODUCTION

Many women (and sometimes even men) tell me that they were so close to giving up on their natural curly hair but after reading my blog and watching my own transitioning journey, it has given them hope that they too can get their curls back.

This was what inspired me to write ALL of my tips and tricks in this book. I too was at a stage with my hair where I just felt like there was nothing I could do to help get it back to health. I was unhappy with my hairs appearance as it was dry, dead and wouldn't curl!

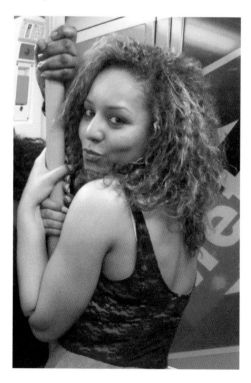

(Summer 2013)

I promise you that if you follow the steps in this book you'll get your hair back to health no matter how damaged it is! This will take time and determination but once you understand the basic principles, the journey will be a fun one, and you will find out what your natural hair likes/dislikes!

I had spent years trying to manipulate my natural hair to be what I 'thought' was acceptable, sitting in salons for hours and hours, spending chunks out of my monthly pay to just damage my hair over and over again.

In 2014 I had reached my breaking point and decided to try out the natural hair journey. I put down the straighteners, stopped my monthly visits to the hair salon, and began to self-teach on how to care for not only my hair but also my self-confidence. I knew that one day I may have my own daughters and how would I be able to care for their hair if I couldn't even manage my own?!

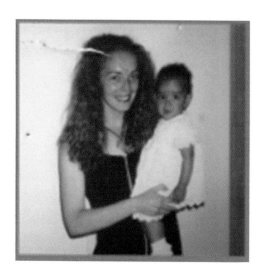

Where it all began..

I was born and bred in South London, United Kingdom, I grew up in the 90's as a mixed race girl (half Scottish, white/half Nigerian, black) around people of all races but few that actually looked like me or had my hair texture. In fact, there were hardly any public figures that embraced their natural curls around that time, long live Scary Spice the original 90's curl icon! I had very low self-confidence when I was a child and HATED any kind of attention or eyes on me. I would literally do anything within my power to avoid being singled out.

My thick curly hair was a part of why I was insecure! My hair had a much tighter curl than the mixed race girls I grew up around and I had enough hair for 3 people! I always felt like I was different and began to hate my hair and the fact that it wouldn't grow down my shoulders and stay the length and smooth texture it was whilst wet. My mum would take care of it by having it in braids most of the time so I rarely had my hair in its natural state growing up.

Back in the late 90's/early 00's in the UK it was a huge struggle for me to find hair products that actually worked well for my hair. I had two choices; curly hair styling products in the UK made for European hair or moisturisers/styler's specifically made for afro/ relaxed hair. There was a visible gap in the market for products that would care for my type of curls.

For years my mum searched for the perfect product, we even researched on what the celebrities were doing! I remember us always wanting to know why it was so hard to find something on the high street. We found that most deep conditioners would make my curls look great but as I couldn't leave them in I just dealt with frizz and thought this was something I would have to live with forever.

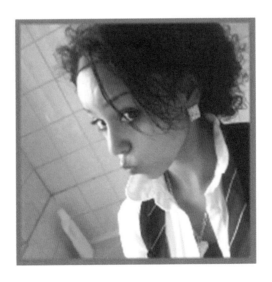

High School

Fast-forward to high school, and I now wanted to be a grown up as you do when you reach your early teens. I decided I was going to take over my own hair care.

With the pressures of puberty, attention from boys, wanting to be an individual in a school full of girls I decided to experiment with my hair colour, and often straightened it to look older (now looking back – my hair was a damn mess!).

My hair is naturally a dark brown colour but I was obsessed with having my hair straight and blonde as that was what most of my favourite singers - that I identified with were doing at that time. Surprisingly later on in life I learnt that it was weaves and wigs they were wearing to have the blonde straight hair I desired.

I compromised with my mum to start with a brown colour and that brown got lighter and lighter as the years went by. I didn't have my natural hair colour from the year 2006 until 2014! Bear in mind most of the time my hair was dyed using the at home kits you buy from the supermarket.

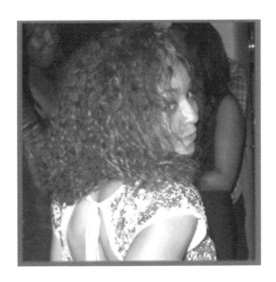

College

The change of hair colour still wasn't good enough for my self-confidence by the time I went to college! College for me was a whole new ball game as I attended the BRIT School for performing arts where many talented people like Adele and Amy Winehouse had went to, so you can imagine how artsy and eccentric people's styles were.

Everyday I was surrounded by many girls of the same race as me (which I hadn't been around before) but again they all had much looser and "easier to manage" curls than I did. I remember envying those that could simply restyle their hair for the rest of the day in the girl's toilets with just water and their hands! I mean I would have needed to bring my whole hair cupboard to do that!

In 2009 towards the end of college, I decided I had had enough of trying to manage my natural hair and wanted looser curls! I was about to move away from London for University and "couldn't deal with managing my hair" anymore, no products were moisturising enough, it would frizz up as soon as my hair dried, and I could never detangle it (sounding familiar?).

After years of begging my mum for a relaxer and her refusing, I took matters into my own hands (as I was grown enough to make my own decisions) and went to a hair stylist who told me that he had two mixed race daughters who had hair textures similar to mine, and relaxed their hair for the same reasons I wanted to.

He sold it to me and I had my hair semi-relaxed (meaning it could be worn both curly and straight), blow-dried, coloured and straightened! This procedure continued every 4-6 months for the next 4 years!

By 2013 I still wasn't over the desire to be blonde and pleaded to take matters into my own hands, despite resistance from my stylist. I went for blonde highlights, and that my friends, was the point of no return! The result was hair that looked like straw, lifeless and dry.

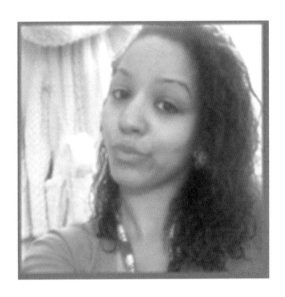

University

Uni was another huge change for me as I moved away from the hustle and bustle of London to Hertfordshire a couple of hours away, of course being away from London had its negatives and I definitely suffered within the hair care department. I couldn't find products for my hair in any of the local stores (there weren't many!) So I found myself stocking up when back in London and continuing to relax my hair just so it would stay low maintenances throughout the three years away from home.

During these 3 years my hair was at it's worst! In my 2nd year of university I actually started a natural hair journey by dyeing my hair back to dark brown and I began moisturising it and putting down the straighteners. This didn't last long and during my final year I decided to take the plunge and go blonde, it was like rebelling!

My Hair Damage Journey in Pictures!

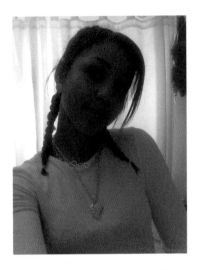

Heat damage (2007)

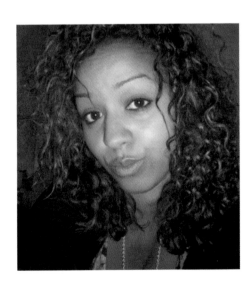

First relaxer (2010)

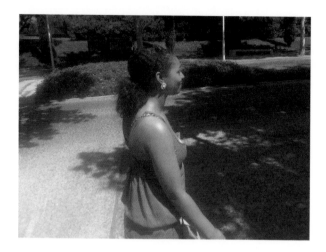

Colour damage (2011)

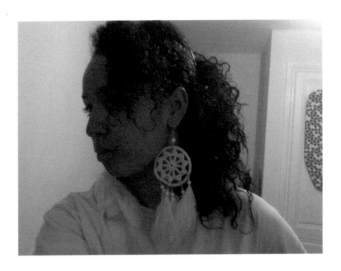

Attempting to transition (2011)

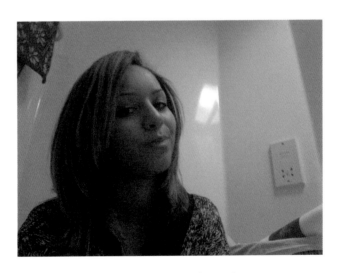

Going Blonde (2012)

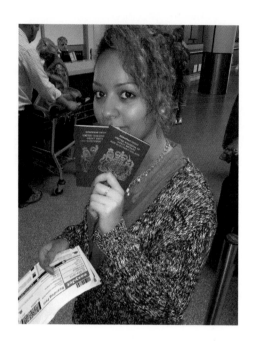

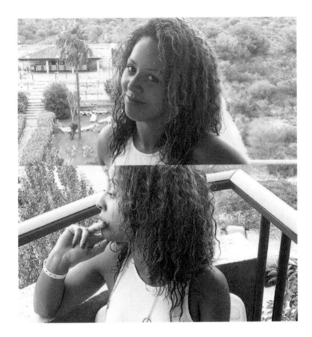

After years of damage, my hair at it's worst! (2013)

So what are your next steps when you have pushed the boat too far? You either give up or keep going, and at that point I was lucky enough to have discovered the amazing 'Natural Hair Community' on YouTube. I began finding so many curly girls sharing their hair routines, and products that I had never even heard of before!

Coconut Oil? Wash and go? Co-wash? I became addicted, it made me so motivated, and confident in the fact that I could maybe turn this around. It took me a year and a piece to get my hair to its natural state, and to the great health that it is today.

Please see me as an example of what NOT to do and as an inspiration that you can turn it around!

MISCONCEPTIONS ABOUT 'GOING NATURAL'

Before we really get into the book I just want to take a moment too reiterate a few points to you all!

Many of us jump the gun when it comes to going natural, or transitioning, and believe in a lot of misconceptions.

"YOU NEED TO"

Everyone's hair is completely different, even if you are the same race or texture, your hair is still going to need, and want different things to others. All we can do in this community is **RECOMMEND & SUGGEST** so do not take everything for gospel; instead do some of your own self-discovery, (I promise you it will be fun and rewarding when you finally get it right!).

"IT'S TOO EXPENSIVE"

This can always be resolved! If you want to go natural but have put it off due to lack of funds, there are cheaper alternatives! Refer to **Chapter 3** for some tips.

"TOO MUCH WORK"

You're right it will take work BUT hold up, you have been trying to maintain your damaged hair and that was hard work too! Now you are just taking matters into your own hands, why deny what you were naturally born with?

Now that we've got that out of the way let's get into the juicy stuff!

By the end of this book I am sure that you will be inspired to start your own natural hair journey, remember this isn't a hair care bible BUT rather some basic principles. The fun is that you will discover what works best for you and what makes your hair truly unique!

2
LET'S GET BACK TO BASICS

What is transitioning?

Transitioning is a process you go through when growing your damaged hair out (for those who don't want to do the 'Big Chop') it can be a lot of work, but also a fun process as you learn more about your natural hair and its rewarding watching your progress! For those who aren't aware this is exactly what I had to do instead of simply cutting off all of my damaged hair.

Whilst transitioning you will be dealing with two or more hair textures, your new natural hair will be growing in and you will still be managing your damaged/straight ends. This takes blending techniques, heavy conditioning and regular treatments to maintain. (We will get into this later!)

Now luckily transitioning to natural hair has been made much easier thanks to many hair care brands, who have created products specifically for transitioners, and hair tools to make natural hair care doable!

QUICK TOP TIPS FOR TRANSITIONING

- Natural ingredients
- No direct heat
- Deep condition with steam/heat
- Protein Treatments
- No harsh tools
- Protective styling

- No more chemicals!

The Line Of Demarcation

The 'Line of demarcation' is something that you will be aware of both before and during your transitioning journey. This is the line where your relaxed/damaged hair meets your natural hair. This line where both types meet is very fragile and prone to breakage so you must make sure you protect and treat it well.

You can protect the line by using strengthening treatments (I will recommend later) and hiding by protective styling.

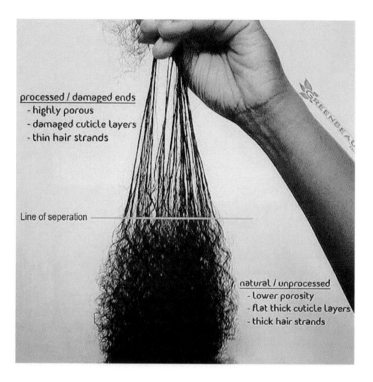

processed / damaged ends
- highly porous
- damaged cuticle layers
- thin hair strands

Line of seperation

natural / unprocessed
- lower porosity
- flat thick cuticle layers
- thick hair strands

http : // naijahaircangrow. blogspot. com/2015/01/ the-line-of-demarcation.html

Hair Typing

Many new naturals feel they need to find out what their hair type is before anything else! However, I am very against hair 'typing' as it seems to create a divide within the community when we should all be celebrating the fact that we are all on the natural hair journey together.

4b, 2a, 3c... I say forget that! Instead find out your hair porosity level (this is where it really gets interesting!) By finding out your hairs porosity level you can then create a full hair regimen suitable for your hair.

What Is Porosity?

Porosity is how well your hair is able to hold and absorb moisture. Your porosity is vital to know about especially as curlies because we are prone to dry hair.

Your hair has cuticles that overlap one another,

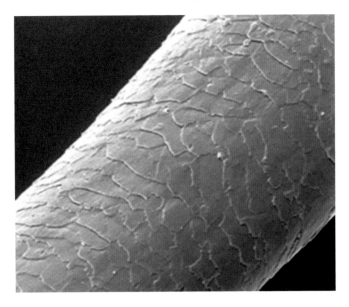

http : // thehairextensionboutique. co. uk/facts/human-hair-structure/

The flexibility of the hair allows oil and moisture into the cuticles, however if your cuticles are tighter this means your hair won't allow in much moisture = low porosity which is what my hair is.

Your hairs porosity level can be affected by heat and chemical processing, which you probably have had if you are reading this. Once you know your hairs porosity (either low, medium or high) you can then begin to understand what techniques and products are likely to work for you.

Here is a quick and easy way to determine your hairs porosity level.   (Bearing in mind that this can change over time.)

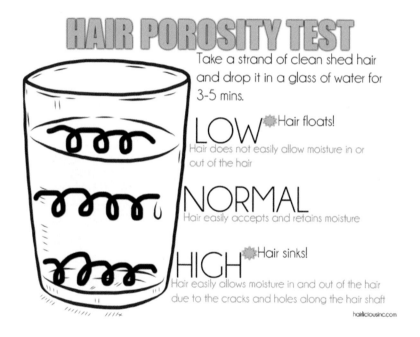

HAIR POROSITY TEST

Take a strand of clean shed hair and drop it in a glass of water for 3-5 mins.

LOW ✸Hair floats!
Hair does not easily allow moisture in or out of the hair

NORMAL
Hair easily accepts and retains moisture

HIGH ✸Hair sinks!
Hair easily allows moisture in and out of the hair due to the cracks and holes along the hair shaft

hairliciousinc.com

Hair Porosity

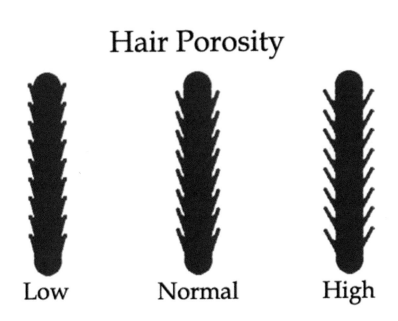

Low   Normal   High

http : // www.african-flair .co .za/healthy-hair-journey/porosity/

TIPS FOR LOW POROSITY

Join the club! Sigh, this is the most difficult level to manage and most probably what you will have as a transitioner, thanks to the damage you have put your hair through. This will make sense as to why you find it a nightmare trying to keep your hair moisturised.

Don't you fear! Here are some tips on how to push that moisture into your stubborn cuticles.

Steam

Just like in-grown hairs and clogged pores steam loosens up the skin and allows the hair to come through the skin. This is perfect for low porosity hair as the steam helps to open the tight cuticles. You can then follow up with a deep conditioner or a leave-in conditioner.

I once went in a steam room with my hair soaked in deep conditioner under a shower cap. AMAZINGLY my hair had never felt so soft I was shocked! Steam will help so much with your dry hair.

If you don't have access to a steam room (which most of us don't) simply steam up your bathroom with the shower or wrap your hair in a shower cap and cover with some warm towels.

Hot Oil Treatments

Lighter oils like Jojoba, Argon and Grapeseed Oil used as a hot oil treatment will also work wonders on your low porosity hair.

Key Products/Ingredients to use

WATER! Aloe Vera, Shea Butter, Raw Honey, Glycerine, Cocoa Butter, and Bentonite Clay.

TIPS FOR MEDIUM POROSITY

Congrats! You will have a much easier ride my friend. Thankfully you aren't at the extremes of either side, which means your hair doesn't need much maintenance. Your cuticles aren't as tight, so will allow in just the right amount of moisture!

This porosity level takes well to heat and colour so you will most likely be able to colour your hair with minimal damage! You should however avoid protein in everyday use and you can deep condition every few weeks or so (up to you!).

Key Products/Ingredients to use

Olive oil, Aloe Vera, Lotions and milks instead of heavier butters.

TIPS FOR HIGH POROSITY

Now this type of porosity is too much of a good thing which equals some curly hair problems! High porosity hair lets in too much moisture which makes it prone to tangling whilst in humidity and frizz. When water hits the hair this can actually cause breakage and damage as the hair absorbs too much! I believe that I must have had high porosity hair as a child, as it was always so frizzy.

To prevent this you need to make sure your hair is sealed, you can do this by layering products e.g. LOC method (liquid, oil and conditioner/cream.) This will help the hair to hold on to the moisture it's given instead of soaking up any more than needed.

Key Products & Ingredients

Protein, Shea Butter, Olive Oil, Aloe Vera, and Apple Cider Vinegar.

Now that you have identified your hairs porosity level, you can use that to your advantage. Try out recommended products, and routines that should work for your hair type. Along with porosity I need you to know all about what ingredients there are out there for you to play with!

Ingredients

On your natural hair journey you will come across a huge range of products to try! Some may work for you, that don't work for others, and vice versa but from my experience I find that products with the majority of their ingredients being natural will transform your hairs health.

Most of the cheapest products you find in the hair shops may have words like "Natural", "Curly", "Coconut", "Olive Oil" written on them BUT unfortunately, they are using the words loosely - all you have to do is take a look at the list of ingredients on the back to find out whether it will be a good choice for your hair or not.

If water/aqua is the first ingredient on the list it is always a pro!

The list of ingredients goes in order of quantities so if Aqua is first it means that the product is made up of mainly water. The first 3-5 ingredients are a great indication of what makes a good product.

For example, I have had friends say to me that they love the results they get from the cheaper products and thought they were made from all natural ingredients due to the packaging but later found out that after a while their hair was breaking and dry. This is due to the lack of great natural moisturising ingredients, which unfortunately is replaced with chemicals in these cheaper products.

Below I have listed a range of products, and their ingredients that are useful to look out for and also a list of ones you should try to avoid!

Natural Gems

Coconut Oil – *Hair Benefits* Reduces protein loss, cools the scalp, amazing conditioner, and a great split end remedy.

Ask any natural/curly haired person on earth what natural products they use on their hair, and I guarantee you that 90% will mention this magical oil! Make sure you only use the 100% pure unrefined coconut oil usually found in health food stores / supermarkets and some hair product stores. This is an oil with multiple uses like most natural ingredients!

Shea Butter – *Hair Benefits* Natural hair protectant, softens the hair, and moisturises.

A great natural cream and alternative if you're ever out of hair products, this will heavily moisturise the hair. When purchasing Shea butter, make sure you get the 100% natural/pure unrefined version, which hasn't been stripped of its natural odour or consistency. Refined Shea butter can have other added ingredients to change its consistency, colour, and odour ridding of the many benefits.

You can find unrefined Shea butter on websites like Amazon or sometimes in local afro hair stores. Unrefined Shea usually smells smoky and comes in hard clumps (similar to a bar of soap) but melts once rubbed in your hands. Shea Butter also has a low level SPF therefore I use it to protect my hair from the sun on holiday.

Olive Oil - *Hair Benefits* Reduces the appearance of dandruff, adds shine, and tames frizz.

Olive Oil coats the outer layer of the hair making it look smooth, it also protects and is perfect as an oil treatment. You will find that it is used lots in the Asian community for skin and hair. I always add virgin olive oil (often my local supermarkets brand) to any hot oil treatment I make.

Jamaican Black Castor Oil - *Hair Benefits* Full of omega-9 fatty acids, vitamin E, it moisturises your roots and promotes hair growth.

A key ingredient used in one of my all-time favourite leave-in conditioners! This is the oil I used a lot during my transitioning stage to help my hair grow and keep my scalp healthy. It also has healing properties that will rid scalp infections, head lice, and dandruff. It is hugely popular as an oil to help grow back your edges, eyebrows and eye lashes.

Aloe Vera - *Hair Benefits* Reduces dandruff, adds shine, and moisturises.

This is one of my summertime favourites to seal my wash and go's. It is great for when you don't have a curl refresher, and I like to apply some on my wet hair. It also helped me a lot when I suffered from a really itchy and irritated scalp.

Jojoba Oil - *Hair Benefits* Unplugs pores in the scalp, rids of oily hair, and promotes growth.

Jojoba oil is actually the oil that is closest to the oil your scalp naturally produces (sebum). This means that if you have an oily scalp, you can apply Jojoba oil and it will trick your skin into balancing the sebum production.

This hair oil is great for hair growth and can actually clear any blockages you may have in your scalp, which in return gives your pores freedom to produce more hair making your hair grow longer. If hair loss is an issue for you – you should definitely incorporate a Jojoba oil scalp massage/application weekly.

Flaxseed Gel – *Hair Benefits* Nourishing, great definition for twist outs, no shedding/breakage, adds shine and moisture.

You may see this ingredient more and more in popular natural hair products as the natural trend gains more popularity, most hair gels are made from flaxseed.

Flaxseeds can be made into a gel at home. You boil the flaxseeds in a pan and stir until the consistency becomes foamy, then you strain and place into a container to cool down. It then becomes gel like in consistency, ready to be applied to the hair (there are tons of step by step, online tutorials on this).

I keep mentioning the benefits for the scalp with all of these oils! This shows you how important scalp care is and how easy it is to look after it naturally!

What to Avoid

Again, please do not take everything I say as gospel, trends change and what works for one head of hair may not work for another. However, the ingredients listed below I feel should be avoided, especially if you are on the road to hair recovery, as you will need all the naturalness and moisture you can get.

Mineral Oil

This is basically the alternative to natural oils, which you will see available in cheaper hair products but in my opinion it is much healthier to use all natural oils than something that can be mass produced.

Mineral oil is derived from crude oil, yes the oil put into cars. When used in hair products the oil is distilled, but when not prepared properly imagine the damage that it can do to your hair when used constantly.

Alcohol

This is an ingredient that I always look out for in any product I buy and like to avoid straight away due to the breakage and dryness it causes! However, after some further research while writing this book, it turns out that there are actually good alcohols and bad alcohols! Here is a list of both the good and the bad used in hair products.

Bad alcohols: Cause dryness and breakage when used frequently.

- SD Alcohol 40

- Ethanol

- SD Alcohol

- Propyl

- Propanol

- Isopropyl

Good alcohols: Used to create the hair products consistency and keeping the oils in the product together.

- Cetyl alcohol

- Stearyl alcohol

- Myristyl alcohol

- Lauryl alcohol

- Behenyl alcohol

- Cetearyl alcohol

Parabens

Parabens are used in cosmetic products as a low cost preservative. You will find them in many of the popular and cheap hair, beauty and skincare products.

However now we are seeing more and more signs on beauty products saying "Free from Parabens" this is because according to recent studies there have been concerns that this ingredient when used on the body overtime, could be a contributor to breast cancer in women.

Sulphates

Sulphates, also written as SLS-sodium lauryl sulphate, ALS-ammonium lauryl sulphate or SLES-sodium lauryl sulphates are chemicals commonly found in cleaning products like soaps and toothpaste.

Sounds crazy that such a harsh chemical used to remove dirt and germs on surfaces are also used to remove the same from your sensitive hair and scalp! Sulphates also create the foam you feel and see when shampooing the hair. Notice how if you get shampoo in your eyes it stings like hell! Yes that is because it is a STRONG chemical that strips your hair, leaving it weak and dry.

You are probably thinking, why are these chemicals even used in hair products? They are used because they are cheap! This means mass production is easier and the products will be available at a more affordable price.

When purchasing products during your transitioning phase try to avoid the above in order to maintain healthy, moisturised hair with a healthy body!

Expiration Date

Have you ever noticed expiry dates on your beauty and hair products? I usually ignore them, as the products always look fine to me, BUT again after doing some research I learnt that the expiry date is actually there for a serious reason! I have products that are around a year old in my cupboard, which I will now throw away and I will explain why.

Most hair products have a shelf life of one year but even this date becomes invalid once the product has been opened, and has had contact with human skin.

Deep conditioners, butters and styling products usually come packaged in a tub where you have to constantly grab the product with your hands. Now imagine the bacteria you are passing into the product AND the water that flows into the tub (if you use in the shower, like I do). This isn't the end of the world at all but just something to think about when it comes to keeping your products fresh.

Conditioners, shampoos and styler's that come in pump bottles are best as nothing can contaminate the product meaning they will last longer. To preserve the product and make sure it stays effective try to keep them away from sunlight and in a cool environment.

After reading this chapter you should now know what transitioning is, have a good idea of your hair type and know what ingredients to use and those to avoid.

3
BALLIN ON A BUDGET (GUIDE TO BUYING PRODUCTS)

A lot of bloggers and influencers are sometimes careful with mentioning products and brands as it may interfere with sponsorship opportunities BUT I have decided that this book is NEEDED and I want to give you all my HONEST opinion and genuine help (even if that means free promotion for the below). Your transformations mean so much more to me!

I must also reinforce that what works for me, another blogger, your friend or neighbour may not necessarily work for you, so please be prepared that you will need to go through your own process. It's usually a case of trial and error with many products/brands until you find your holy grails.

EASILY ACCESIBLE BRANDS

I am speaking from a UK perspective as many of the below products have been available in the USA way before the UK. These are brands I feel are great and are available in most of the natural/afro hair shops in the UK, and now mainstream stores on the high streets of London and around the UK.

I live in South London and find that Brixton has an amazing selection of afro hair stores, stocking the best UK and USA natural hair brands, usually found surrounding the market area.

Here are some of the brands you will find around that I recommend,

Cantu – Made with 100% pure Shea Butter, and no harsh chemicals.

Cantu was one of the first brands I found that actually styled and moisturised my hair. It has such an amazing smell and I always get comments about the scent when I have these products in my hair. I always point people towards Cantu as an alternative to the more expensive natural hair care brands. Although, it isn't 100% natural, if you have no problems with this and just want something affordable and a product that will provide moisture, then you can use Cantu as your starting point.

Each product typically costs: Under £10

Key ingredients: Shea Butter, Jojoba Oil, and Sweet Almond Oil.

My favourites are: Conditioning Treatment Masque, Leave in conditioner and Coconut Curling Cream.

CURLS – No sulphates, silicones, parabens or mineral oil.

This is a very popular brand in the natural hair world! CURLS have all types of products to meet your needs and they all include natural ingredients. The products are a bit more expensive over here in the UK but recommended especially for styling. I love the smells and vibrant packaging!

Each product typically costs: £8 - £19

Key ingredients: Aloe Vera, Shea Butter, Glycerine, and Grape Seed Oil.

My favourites are: *Curl Curlada Conditioner, and Crème Brule Whipped   Curl Cream.*

Shea Moisture – Natural Shea Butter, organic and cruelty free.

If you know me you will get sick of me going on and on about this brand, but I can't get enough. I fell in love with these products at the start of my natural hair journey after watching tutorials and reviews from YouTubers like HeyFranHey and SunKissAlba! This brand right here is the first brand that actually was able to style, manage and moisturise my hair, long term, not just for the first few hours!

I definitely recommend it and they now have so many ranges for different hair types so you are bound to find something that works for you.

The products are also available in Boots and Superdrug for my UK readers. My favourite range is the Jamaican Black Castor Oil collection.

Each product typically costs: £9.99 - £12.99

Key ingredients: Shea Butter, Coconut Oil, and Jamaican Black Castor Oil.

My favourites are: Jamaican Black Castor Oil Strengthen & Restore Leave-in Conditioner, Super fruit Complex 10-in-1 Treatment Masque, and Jamaican Black Castor Oil Shampoo.

AsIAm – Organic ingredients with no harsh chemicals.

A brand that became available in the local afro hair shops a few years ago. I tried the Coconut Co-wash and fell in love instantly! It smells amazing, comes in a great sized tub so you can apply generously to detangle and co-wash. It leaves the hair feeling so fresh and detangled thanks to the great slip and moisture.

Each product typically costs: £9.99 - £18

Key ingredients: Coconut Oil, Tangerine Extract, and Castor Oil.

My favourites are: Coconut Co-wash and Cleansing Conditioning.

ApHogee – Cruelty free, Uses proteins, amino acids, emollients and humectants to restore hair.

An important brand for you to explore when you first start your journey! All products are very strong and get rid of the damage effectively. They have systems that are used in salons so you MUST read the instructions and even watch some tutorials on how to use them before trying for yourself.

Each product typically costs: £4 - £10

Key ingredients: Keratin, Protein and Amino Acids.

My favourites are: Two-Step Protein Treatment, and Keratin 2 Minute Reconstructor.

ECOco – Naturally derived ingredients, moisture and hold.

The styler gel from this brand changed the game for me! This gel is the ONLY gel that will actually slick my hair down and make it stay! This was always an issue for me growing up as I always found its gets flaky, dries the hair, smells unpleasant, or would not make the hair stay in place and this was such a difficulty! The gels come in different sized tubs and different options of oils.

Each product typically costs: Under £5

Key ingredients: Olive Oil, Wheat Protein and Glycerine.

My favourites are: Olive Oil Eco Styler Gel and the Argon Oil Eco Styler Gel.

Sunny Isle - This brand is the creator of some amazing oils organically grown in Jamaica, which moisturise and help the hair to grow. I like that the brand has mixed different scents with the Jamaican Black Castor Oil as it naturally has a real smoky scent which isn't nice at all.

Each product typically costs: £3.99 - £10

Key ingredients: Jamaican Castor Oil and Coconut Oil.

My favourites are: Lavender Jamaican Black Castor Oil.

UK Natural Hair Brands

Here in the UK we also have a great range of home-grown brands selling 100% natural and organic hair products. Check out some of my favourites below.

Big Hair – This natural hair brand includes no nasty chemicals encouraging us all to wear our hair big and proud!

Each product typically costs: £9.96 - £15

Key Ingredients: Aloe Vera Juice, Shea Butter, Coconut Oil, and Sweet Almond Oil.

My Favourites are: *Moisture Me Whipped Hair Butter, and Deep Conditioning Hair Treatment.*

Root2Tip – Provides natural products that really focus on growing and maintaining the hair's health.

Each product typically costs: £10 - £13.99

Key ingredients: Castor Oil, Rosemary, Lavender, and Coconut Oil.

My favourites are: *Grow It Long Scalp Serum.*

Boucleme – One of my favourite brands! Great products with a citrus scent and natural ingredients which are amazing for styling curls.

Each product typically costs: £15 - £19

Key ingredients: Glycerine, Coconut Oil, Argon Oil, Kukui Oil, and Shea Butter.

My favourites are: *Curl Cream and Curl Conditioner.*

Trepadora – Rainforest inspired with beautiful packaging, naturally derived, and vegan!

Each product typically costs: £9 - £19

Key ingredients: Acai Berry, Papaya and Avocado.

My favourites are: *Coconut Almond Smoothing Conditioner, Papaya Slip and Taming Potion.*

Curly Ellie – For curly kids! Created to make styling your child's curls easier and healthier for both you and them.

Each product typically costs: £12.99 - £14.99

Key ingredients: Aloe Vera, Seed Oil's and Almond Oil.

My favourite is: *Gentle Shampoo*

(The prices mentioned above are relevant to the time of writing this book and are subject to change)

For those on a budget?

I know that back when I was a student I was on a very tight budget, and haircare products were too expensive! I often opted for alternatives like making my own products. Below you will find some useful hacks.

DIY Conditioners

Coconut oil – You can get large jars of 100% natural coconut oil and get so many uses out of it! It can be your pre-poo, scalp treatment, deep conditioner and leave-in.

Shea Butter – Again you can also purchase this in a large package for cheap and use it as a hair and body moisturiser.

Aloe Vera – Aloe Vera was a great curl refresher for me when I was on a tight budget, its consistency is water based so perfect for when you don't want to re-soak your hair when styling.

Flaxseed Gel – You can cook flaxseeds to make a 100% natural hair gel! Gives great definition and shine. Can be made at home like I mentioned in Chapter 1.

DIY Treatments

Protein treatment – Egg (make sure you DO NOT warm up), mayonnaise, natural yoghurt all help to strengthen the hair.

Hot Oil treatment – Jojoba Oil, Jamaican Black Castor Oil, Almond Oil, Peppermint Oil, Coconut Oil (most moisturising oils!) all mixed together will give your scalp and hair a great deep moisture treatment.

Deep conditioning treatment – Honey, Olive Oil, Coconut Oil, Almond Oil, Castor Oil, Avocado and Banana are all amazing ingredients to blend together and soak your hair for some moisture.

After reading this chapter you should know what products are out there for you to try, and what you can do when you're on a tight budget (No excuses!).

4
HAIR TUTORIALS & CHILL

So you have your hair type and a choice of great products/brands to begin using. NOW you want to get started with the styling and the beginning of your transitioning journey! But where exactly do you start?

When I embarked on my journey I spent about a week watching different curly hair routines on YouTube and advice from blogs about 'How to wash curly hair, curly hair routines, natural hair journeys', and more. This really helped to inspire me, gave me great demonstrations, and evidence that the journey works.

The Internet is your oyster, all you have to do is type in any search engine **"curly hair"** and you will have days' worth of "how to's", "tutorials", "product reviews", "top tips/advice", and more!

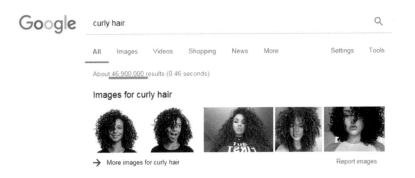

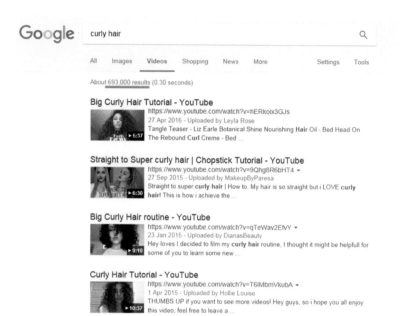

Start by clicking on videos where the person has a similar hair type as yours (from looking at them) gather some of your favourites and notice what techniques or products they all seem to have in common. For example, I realised that girls with similar hair to mine would style their hair whilst it was soaking wet, then apply product and detangle with their fingers.

Soon you will feel confident enough try the routines out on your next washday! The first one is always an exciting one but don't get disheartened if you fail (Girrlll I had so many major fails but this is how you become a pro!) and you might even be inspired to make your own channel.

After reading this chapter you will have probably watched hours of videos online and may have become a hair tutorial addict but its ok! Let's get back to your journey!

5
HAIR DETOX

Now you have the proof and all the tools you need to start, like you would do when starting a new diet you want to get rid of anything that is unhealthy for your hair, start by staying away from **heat** (this is the best tip) as heat is such a major setback. Each time you apply straighteners, hot combs or hot blow dryers to the hair you are damaging the hair shaft and gradually training your curls to be straight!

You may find that your new routine may not be working as fast as you wish, but I promise you – you will find no REAL improvement in your hairs health or length unless you are patient and stop being a slave to the straighteners!

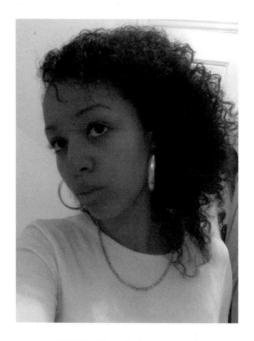

2007 (Heat damage)

What is heat damage?

Heat damage is when your curls are no longer their natural texture due to constant heat tools drying out and straightening the hair so much that it loses its curl even after washing. Years of damage will leave you with limp, dry hair with no elasticity.

I have heard these stories over and over again,

"My hair was looking amazing! But then I had an event so I straightened my hair and now after washing, it just isn't the same!!"

"I now have straggly straight parts of my hair after straightening it just one time!"

Don't let this be you, if you are going to go back to heat I recommend doing it once your hair has fully recovered and is healthy and natural. Make sure you use the correct heat protection, and treatments before and after.

What is colour damage?

Something I again abused over my teenage years! Constantly using hair dyes and heat like I mentioned above will eventually lead to dry hair and often your hair will break off (especially if you are lightening your hair or bleaching it blonde). This is referred to as colour damage. Luckily, there are now much safer ways to colour your curly hair, particularly as our hair is prone to dryness.

During the transitioning phase your hair is very sensitive so I would avoid colouring your hair at all costs during this stage.

I found this part difficult as not only was I transitioning from heat/chemical damage, I also had blonde hair that I had to grow out, which did not match my natural hair colour growing through.

Each to their own, but if you feel more comfortable dying your hair back to its natural colour and then transitioning, make sure you go down the safe route and use an expert.

Here are some alternatives and safer ways to colour your hair if you are not convinced…

- Hair Chalk

- Henna
- Honey Colour
- Hair Colour Rinse

What is chemical damage?

Chemical damage is the terrible effects relaxers, texturisers, straightening systems, Brazilian blowouts, and perms do to the hair.

Remember I semi-relaxed my hair every 6-9 months for 5 years straight because I wanted a looser curl that was 'easy to manage'. This resulted in thinning, straight, dry, shedding hair. All of the hair treatments I mentioned above include harsh chemicals that are damaging to the hair and your body.

Have you noticed that they can only be applied for a certain amount of time? That is due to how dangerous they can be if left on for longer. I have felt the burn a relaxer can give to the scalp when you leave it in for too long and that is not a good sign!

Quick Breakdown of Chemical Treatments

Relaxers

Also known as "Creamy crack", are a 'controlled' way to damage the protein structure of your hair (KEYWORD:

DAMAGE) this results in looser waves/curls or if wanted can turn your hair completely straight.

If you are reading this, I am pretty sure that you know relaxers aren't good for your hairs health but they are also not good for your body. The scalp can suffer severe chemical burns if over exposed to lye or no-lye relaxers.

Hair relaxers were 'the' hair revolution back in 1877, which in my opinion is sort of an underlying slave mentality that we all may have inside, whether we really know it or not, but we desire the same hair type as our European sisters.

With lye

Relaxers that have NO LYE consist of the chemical Sodium Hydroxide (sounds scary right?) mixed with water, petroleum jelly, mineral oil, and emulsifiers to create a creamy consistency to apply easily to the hair.

No lye

You will find other relaxers that have the slogan 'No Lye' which means it isn't as harsh and includes a weaker chemical like 'Potassium hydroxide, lithium hydroxide, or guanidine hydroxide. No Lye is becoming the more popular option but it still isn't the way to go!

Brazilian Blow out

This has become popular over the last 10 years or so, mostly popular within Dominican hair salons and seen as a better way of straightening the hair for those with wavy hair. It leaves the hair dead straight, no frizz, bounce and shine. You get all of this with just using a blow-dryer.

Keratin Treatment

This is a way of straightening the hair with frizz free results lasting around 2 months. The Keratin product is applied to the hair and then your hair is straightened to seal. In the salon you are guaranteed no damage that is if they use the correct tools. Brazilian blowouts are similar but just use a blow-dryer, however the chemicals included like 'Formaldehyde' cause long-term damage!

Straightening Strengthening Systems

This is a newer product on the market that a lot of the leading black hair brands are creating. The ORS Straightening and Strengthening Treatment is said to last 4-6 weeks before your hair reverts to its original texture. This type of treatment is aimed at naturals as a way to straighten their hair, and revert it back to its natural state without using a relaxer.

I myself have watched many girls review these products and show that it still damaged the hair so I am sceptical about these systems. I recommend reading/watching many reviews yourself before going ahead with using one!

As you can see all of the above treatments lead to some kind of damage and increase damage to your scalp! Cutting out all of the above is going to give your hair the care it needs.

As you will find out over the next few months your hair will be getting a lot stronger and like everything in life the longer you stick to it the more your new haircare routine will become second nature. I haven't straightened my hair since 2013! That comes from someone who would have straightened at least once a month.

How To Repair Your Hair

"Out with the old and in with the new!"

Getting rid of all the bad habits you have when dealing with your hair, leaves room for new products and routine that will begin to fix the damage. Along with growing out your damaged hair, there are ways to repair it whilst going through the process. It's no good just leaving it to grow our without treating it along the way for that extra push.

Treatments

I am a HUGE advocate for weekly treatments, this definitely transformed my hairs health and if planned out right you will see changes very fast! Damaged and dead hair needs moisture and protein to strengthen and grow. I would start your transitioning journey off to a great start by using a protein treatment. Protein treatments penetrate the hairs cortex and are able to fill in any gaps in the cuticle ultimately repairing dead, split hair in the process strengthening the hair also.

You can make your own protein treatments at home by mixing raw eggs (DO NOT rinse with warm water, you may create scrambled eggs in your curls lol), mayonnaise and avocado.

If you are confident enough, research into the correct way to apply the 'Aphogee Two-Step Protein Treatment' as this is a much more intense treatment (meant for professional use) so please read the instructions thoroughly. This treatment will do a great job of fixing the most damaged of hair.

Once you have completed the protein treatment you should see a difference in your hairs health. From then on only perform this treatment again every 6 weeks as it is very strong and if misused could actually cause more damage to your hair.

I used this product twice out of my 2-3 year transitioning journey. Once I saw a difference in healthy I swapped to a weaker treatment like the 'Aphogee Keratin 2 Minute Reconstructor' or ' Crece Pelo Natural Phitoterapeutic Treatment' which straight away you'll see your curls bounce back!

In between protein/keratin treatments you MUST deep condition weekly, skipping these treatments is out of the question if you want to fix your hair. Deep conditioning treatments will train your hair to retain moisture and keep it intact for the week ahead. I find that when I skip deep conditioning on wash day, my hair has more frizz, is dryer and harder to detangle or manage throughout the week.

Scalp Treatments

The last treatment to introduce is scalp treatments, which are particularly important in the beginning stages of your journey to get your hair to grow faster. All you have to do is mix some oils together (be sure to include a drop or 2 or peppermint essential oil) to stimulate the scalp get the blood flowing and start producing hair! I like to warm up my oil mix and massage it into my scalp for 5-10 minute and then wash out.

After reading this chapter you will know what to cut out forever and what to start introducing in order to repair your hair! Hard work pays off, look at it as an investment and healthy hair will be the outcome.

6
HOW TO WASH YOUR CURLS

Here are all the important steps to washing curly hair. Your wash routine will most likely change when you begin to transition, new products and a new way of doing things will have to be introduced to get the best results! Curly hair is so complex and needs to be treated carefully. Once you follow the steps below you will see a complete difference in your hair.

When I began my natural hair journey, I discovered how beneficial deep conditioning weekly is for your hair's health is. Prior to this, I would deep condition at the best monthly but at one point only when I attended the hairdressers!

Deep Conditioning

If you have ever had a deep conditioning treatment at a hair salon you will remember how soft and amazing your hair feels after, now imagine if you keep this up weekly how much your hair's health will improve.

Detangling

Along with weekly deep conditioning you will also want to adopt a new technique of detangling your hair. To prevent damage at the start of my journey I began to finger detangle my curls which means using your fingers as a comb and working through the knots from your ends to your roots (ONLY do this on wet and saturated in conditioner hair). This gentle way of detangling is going to keep your line of demarcation intact and you will start to notice less shedding.

If after a few try's you don't like to finger detangle, try a wide tooth comb as it will act in a similar way, as long as you stay away from fine tooth combs and even the beloved Denman brush at the start of your journey for the best results.

Product

When washing curly hair you shouldn't be afraid when it comes to product measurements, when it comes to co-washing, I apply a very generous amount of product as it just helps to get through the hair for each detangling (Remember curly hair is much dryer so needs more product). I also use this principle when it comes to my leave-in conditioner on day one, meaning that I don't have to reapply product until day 3 or 4. I adopted this routine and saw an improvement in my curls moisture retention and definition.

QUICK TOP TIPS FOR WASH DAY

- Weekly Deep Conditioning
- Finger detangling/Use a wide tooth comb
- Use plenty of conditioner
- Keep your hair wet whilst styling
- Never dry with a bath towel (Use a T-shirt or microfiber towel)

My Typical Wash Day

STEP 1

I like to shampoo/cleanse my hair (due to my scalp) whilst in the shower as I find it easier on my neck and easier to keep my hair saturated at all times. I start by completely soaking my hair in the lukewarm water and then gather a handful of shampoo/cleanser (WITHOUT

Sulphates & Parabens) and begin to massage the product into my scalp only, YES gone are the days of scrubbing all the way down to the ends, this completely dries out the hair.

The product when rinsed out naturally cleans the length of the hair without you overdoing it! Once I feel like my scalp is clean I will make sure my hair is still wet (As it is easier to style and detangle whilst wet.) I then get out of the shower wrap myself in a towel and put an old t-shirt around my shoulders to protect my skin from the product I am about to apply (This also saves my hair from the frizz that a usual towel creates.)

STEP 2

Next I go in with my treatment which will usually be a bought deep conditioner with natural ingredients like the Shea Moisture 'Manuka Honey & Mafura Oil Intensive Hydration Masque' apply this in sections (usually 4)

generously! I mean so generous that you can see the product in your hair.

STEP 3

Now you want to cover with a shower cap (I usually grab a plastic bag from around the house). You can leave your hair like this for half an hour. I used to believe longer than an hour would benefit you but actually around the 30-45minute mark, the product will start to seep out of the hair and it becomes pointless.)

To gain maximum results you should apply some heat during this process whether that is with a hooded dryer, thermal cap, steamer or warm towels. I like to use a thermal cap that warms up in the microwave for convenience.

STEP 4

Once your hair has been deep conditioned you can rinse out, I like to use cool water to prevent frizz for when I style next.

Once my hair is completely rinsed I then keep my hair soaking wet (this helps get maximum results from your wash and go styling products)

If you prefer to style dry/damp hair cover with a t-shirt and squeeze out the excess water.

STEP 5

Now my favourite part; first I apply a very light water based leave-in conditioner with great slip 'SheaMoisture Jamaican Black Castor Oil Leave-in', 'Tresemme Naturals conditioner', 'Kinky Curly Knot Today' in sections.

With each section I apply the product to the hair until it feels slippery and stretched. Next I start the detangling process which should be much easier as you have deep conditioned and moisturised. I like to use my fingers for this and grip the hair with one hand at the middle of the length and with the other hand begin detangling from the bottom upwards until I can rake my fingers through my hair from root to tip with no tangles. Once all sections are detangled I like to finish off with a curling cream or gel to get the curl definition I love!

When applying the styling product 'Boucleme Curl Cream' I apply a dime sized amount and smooth through the section this is to prevent product build up and not interrupt the curl pattern.

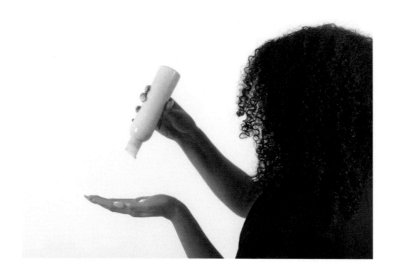

STEP 6

Time to air-dry, I like to leave my hair once styled to air dry (meaning no hair dryers or towels) you do not want to touch your hair during this process as it will interrupt and cause frizz. Depending on the weather this usually takes around 1-2 hours to be bone dry. Once my hair is dry it does shrink up, shrinkage is healthy! It means that your hair has great elasticity (a sign of healthy hair).

Now you know my typical wash day routine! Check out next an example of a regimen you can follow.

7
REGIMEN

This chapter is probably one of the most important chapters for beginners.

You've identified what you need to cut out of your routine, your hair type and what great products/ingredients you should use. Now it's time to create a regimen that works for you!

Your hair care regimen is going to change a lot in the beginning stages of your transition, as you'll be trying out many different products and techniques but try not to obsess and become what they call a "product junkie". It's easy to get caught up in buying all of the new products and trying out every brand like I did in the early stages but it can cost a lot.

I spent around 25% of my pay cheque per month on new products that I didn't need! This isn't necessary, once you find what works for you stick to it until it is completely finished and then re-up on what you like or try something new.

The products I use for my routine often change but below are a list of my staples.

Products for My Wash & Go's

- Shea Moisture JBCO leave-in
- Boucleme Conditioner

- Boucleme Curl Cream
- Boucleme Gel
- Shea Moisture Jamaican Black Castor Oil Shampoo

Products for Twist out's, Braid out's, Bantu Knots

- Big Hair Moisture Me Butter
- Hydratherma Naturals Aloe Curl Enhancing Twisting Cream

Products for No Heat Styling (Curlformers, Perm Rods, Flexi-Rods.)

- Olive Oil Mousse/Set lotion
- Shea Moisture Curl Enhancing Smoothie

Products for Deep Conditioning/Treatments

- Shea Moisture Super Fruit Complex 10 in 1 Treatment Masque
- Crece Pelo Natural Phitoterapeutic Treatment
- Aphogee 2 Minute Keratin Reconstructor
- Root 2 Tip Scalp Serum

I'm going to take you through a basic example of my routine day by day throughout a month.

My Monthly Hair Regimen Example

WEEK 1:

SUNDAY (WASH DAY)

- Oil Massage, Cleanse, Protein Treatment, Deep Condition, Rinse and Wash & go.
- Sleep with hair in a pineapple, satin scarf and satin pillowcase.

MONDAY

- Lightly spritz with water any undefined curls.
- Sleep with hair in a pineapple, satin scarf and satin pillowcase.

TUESDAY

- Style hair in a pineapple, Apply conditioner to my edges to neaten up.
- Sleep with hair in a pineapple, satin scarf and satin pillowcase.

WEDNESDAY

- Co-wash in the shower
- Wash and go using a leave-in conditioner and cream. (Diffuse if cold weather)
- Sleep with hair in a pineapple, satin scarf and satin pillowcase.

THURSDAY

- Spritz with water/light conditioner OR style into a pineapple or bun.

- Sleep with hair in a pineapple, satin scarf and satin pillowcase.

FRIDAY

- Dampen the hair add some conditioner and restyle the up do with some gel.
- Sleep with hair in a pineapple, satin scarf and satin pillowcase.

SATURDAY/SUNDAY

- Cleanse, Deep Condition, Style (Wash and go), Air-dry.
- Sleep with hair in a pineapple, satin scarf and satin pillowcase.

WEEK 2:

MONDAY

- Fluff curls after yesterdays wash & go
- Sleep with hair in a pineapple, satin scarf and satin pillowcase.

TUESDAY

- Style hair in a pineapple, apply some leave-in conditioner if needed.
- Sleep with hair in a pineapple, satin scarf and satin pillowcase.

WEDNESDAY

- Re style hair into a high bun, applying some product to edges and sleeking with a slick/hard bristle brush.
- Sleep with hair in a pineapple, satin scarf and satin pillowcase.

THURSDAY

- Co-wash and style curls (wash and go), air dry.
- Sleep with hair in a pineapple, satin scarf and satin pillowcase.

FRIDAY

- Fluff or refresh curls (Using water and some product)

- Sleep with hair in a pineapple, satin scarf and satin pillowcase.

SATURDAY/SUNDAY

- Cleanse, Deep Condition and Style (Twist out/Braid out), Air Dry or Hooded Dryer.
- Cover hair with a satin scarf and satin pillowcase.

You can apply a braid out or bantu knots instead of a twist out. (Whatever your preference is).

WEEK 3: Twist out/Braid out

MONDAY

- Maintain the twist-out by only unravelling twists when they are fully dry
- Sleep with hair in a pineapple, satin scarf and satin pillowcase.

TUESDAY

- Add some oil to hair if the twist out is dry
- Sleep with hair in a pineapple, satin scarf and satin pillowcase.

WEDNESDAY

- Re style the twist out into an updo
- Sleep with hair in a pineapple, satin scarf and satin pillowcase.

THURSDAY

- Co-wash if needed
- Sleep with hair in a pineapple, satin scarf and satin pillowcase.

FRIDAY

- Pineapple

- Sleep with hair in a pineapple, satin scarf and satin pillowcase.

SATURDAY/SUNDAY

- Cleanse, Deep Condition and Style
- Cover hair with a satin scarf and satin pillowcase.

WEEK 4: (REPEAT WEEK 1)

Each month I alternate depending on my mood, I will either do a scalp oil treatment or a protein treatment, as my hair is no longer damaged. For newly transitioners I recommend using a protein treatment monthly until you see an improvement in your hairs health.

This is an example of what I would do with my hair for a typical month but as you know, this can change depending on the weather, life events, and mood.

After reading this chapter make a hair diary or even add notes on your phone with the things that work best for your hair and anything that doesn't. Set reminders of when to wash your hair, and get your 4-6 week protein treatments in.

8
WHATEVER THE WEATHER

The regimen I have mentioned above will give you a great idea of where to start with your hair care routine, but things can change with the weather like everything in life!

In the UK we hardly have really humid weather, but when I do travel to hot countries I notice that my hair routine has to switch up in order for my hair to stay moisturised.

Below are some of the things you should introduce into your routines during certain seasons.

Spring/Summer Hair Care

Humidity is like marmite you either love it or hate it! Me personally I enjoy humidity I feel products work best for me in this type of climate, and that could be due to the fact that my hair has low porosity.

However, some curlies hate humidity as it causes instant frizz!

To keep your hair protected from the sun you can use natural sun protectants like Coconut Oil, Avocado Oil and Shea Butter.

Whilst on trips to Florida over the past few years I have noticed that I have to co-wash my hair EVERYDAY due to the sweat. Shampoo will often make my scalp really dry so I often co-wash in the mornings whilst in the shower to moisturise and refresh my curls, then a deep conditioner every few days.

I love to rock my hair crazy in the summer for those sunny selfies but as we know our hair dries out quicker in the sun, so you can leave the house with wet hair (always a bonus when you want to save styling time).

Autumn/Winter Hair Care

This season is when it gets a bit more complicated, you have to make sure you keep that hair in order! For me scalp care is a must during the colder months, I naturally get an itchy and dry scalp (my mother does too so I blame her!) so hot oil treatments and occasional oiling of the scalp is a must for me during the winter months.

You may want to explore the LOC/LCO methods, which is washing your hair then styling it in 3 steps,

1. Applying L (Liquid) often water or a water based product, watered down product.
2. Applying O (Oil) to penetrate the hair and give your hair the moisturising benefits it needs.
3. Applying C (Cream) often Shea Butter or a hair butter, thicker moisturiser to add a thicker layer of moisture to seal the first 2 steps in.

The last 2 steps can be switched around depending on what your hair prefers.

My hair prefers the LCO method. These steps will give your hair the extra TLC it needs to get through the cold dryer months.

You can also play with styles that will keep in the moisture like buns, top knots, or have your hair tucked away in a turban/head wrap and more.

Protective Styling

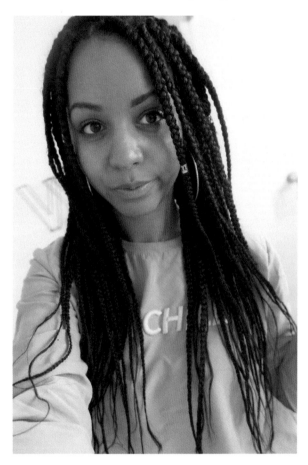

This is a hugely popular solution to winter! Installing braids, twists and more with extensions are a great way to tuck away your natural hair and protect it from the cold. It also gives you a break from having to do your hair everyday (It can be harder in the winter as you will want your hair to be dry when facing any cold weather to avoid colds.

A great benefit to wearing protective styles is that your hair will also have the time and space to grow (which is what we want to happen when transitioning) you will also be able to hide the 2 different textures you may have.

After reading this chapter you should be prepared to take any season by storm!

9

EMBRACE THE MESS 'Twists & Braids & Coils, Oh My!'

So many curlies come to me with the same concern when considering transitioning and that is 'What do I do with my hair whilst it is in this state!'

During your transitioning journey there will be stages when you want to give up, as to be honest your hair may not look exactly how you want it to look when you wear it out. Wash and go's aren't often an option at this stage due to the two different curl patterns (Your old straight/damaged hair and your new natural curls).

The two together do not match but fear not, here are some ways you can combat this stage and fall in love with your hair without giving up. It definitely helped me get through the journey.

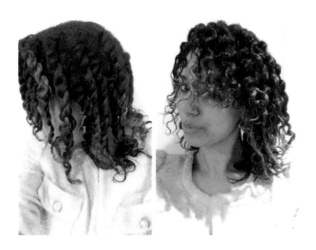

Twist out

This is probably one of the easiest of protective styling/transitioning hairstyles. The results (when done properly) are amazing uniform curls. This is one of the first styles I mastered when transitioning, like everything it takes trial and error. But once you know your hairs porosity you can also skip more epic fails as you will know what products and ingredients will work best for you.

I get the best twist outs when I use a leave-in conditioner and seal with a butter or thicker curl cream. I don't get great results if this is done on dry hair and I have to make sure my twists are 100% dry before taking them out to get the perfect twist out!

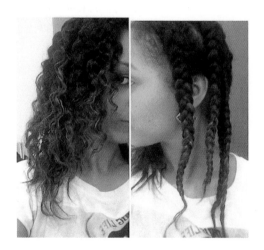

Braid out

Similar results as a twist out, but just even more definition. I bet you have created a braid out before (even without knowing it!) I used to have braid outs all the time as a child, my hair would always be in braids so when taken down I would have perfect uniformed waves, which is basically a braid out! If you can plait this will be an easy task for you, but if you can't you may want to stick with thicker plaits (e.g. 2 on each side of the hair), they don't have to be cornrows/French braids.

Now when it comes to braid outs I actually prefer to do them on an old wash and go as I like to create them when my hair is dry and using some hair butter or even just coconut oil to leave in overnight.

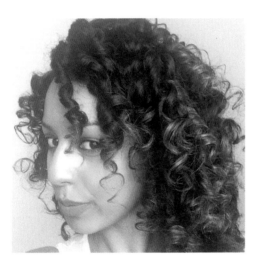

Curl-formers

Curl-formers are a tool that transforms your curls with no heat! You literally end up with hair that looks like it's been curled with a heat tool. All you do is slip the hair through the Curl-former with a hook (don't worry you won't pull your hair out) let it air-dry or use a hood dryer, slip the Curl-formers off and your hair will be so sleek, and in a curl pattern of your choice.

Perm rods

Perm rods are great for creating an afro look especially for those transitioning with shorter hair, this no heat style will be perfect for you to switch up the style! Similar to most of these styles you will start with wet hair, apply product, then section the hair and wind the perm rod around the hair. Roll out the rods once your hair is completely dry.

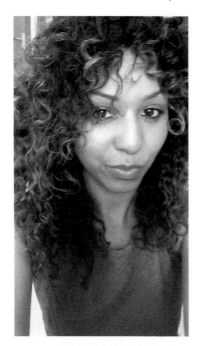

Flexi-rods

Similar to the perm rod style but are a softer almost foam like material. If perm rods aren't for you due to your hairs length, flexi-rods may be a better option. They come in different lengths and thickness's to give different results.

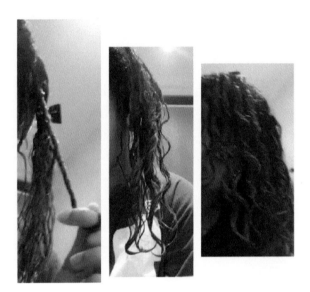

Finger coils

This technique creates the "Shirley Temple" style curls. You create this look by simply curling the hair section by section around your finger. You need products with great hold for this, I personally like to use a curling cream like the Hydratherma Naturals Aloe Curl Enhancing Twisting Cream to get the right grip without leaving the hair dry. This can take a long time to achieve but nice if you want a break as you can separate the coils day by day to get more volume.

Protective styling

If you feel like the above styles are too difficult or time consuming during your transitioning period you can simply turn to protective styles which are wigs, weave, box braids, crotchet braids and twists. These are great if applied and looked after properly, try not to apply too much pressure to the hair, as it is sensitive and you do want your hair to grow! Also make sure you are still washing and treating your scalp.

All of these tools are going to come in handy when you're transitioning. We all want our hair to look good and acceptable, especially so when you're dealing with the driest and deadest of hair. If you use these tools along with great products you can still have your hair looking brand new!

After reading this chapter you are all set for the, "I can't do this" days!

10
HOW TO MAKE IT GROW!

Now it's time to grow the damaged hair out! It took me one and a half-year until I felt ready to cut my hair as it was at a length I was comfortable with! My hair has grown from above shoulder length to bra strap length in one year! This is the most I have ever seen my hair grow (I honestly had come to terms with the fact that my hair would never be long). Oh how wrong I was!

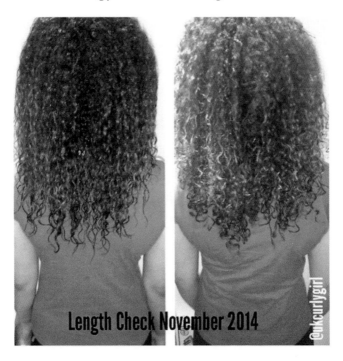

Now all of the past chapters are going to contribute to your hair growth but I will mention below my top 3 hair growth tips that worked well for me, and are the main reasons why my hair has grown so much.

Nurture the scalp

It all begins with the scalp; this is where your hair grows from, so caring for the scalp should be a big priority for you if longer hair is what you desire. One of the main reasons why people find that their hair growth is stunted is because they suffer from product build up and blocked follicles!

This can be easily solved by properly cleansing the scalp weekly and giving it a massage or even scalp scrub every so often. I try and do an oil treatment every other week.

Natural Ingredients

Make your hair grow by using certain special ingredients! There are specific oils that can be used on the scalp to stimulate it (causing hair growth to speed up). Oils like Jamaican Black Castor Oil, and Jojoba Oil are good for this. I would recommend weekly scalp massages using one of the oils above or a hair product with a mix of oils to promote hair growth.

Healthy Eating

I have been a vegetarian/vegan (I am still finding it hard to cut out cheese!, Ok), since January 2015, which was a HUGE adjustment for me (as I used to LOVE meat, burgers, chicken it all!) Due to health reasons and after watching a few documentaries on health I took the step to cut out meat all together and try a healthier diet.

Along with a healthier diet I also now drink a lot more water, at least 2 litres a day. I feel this has helped my hair grow and I have seen a big difference in my eyelashes and eyebrow growth. I used to be able to get at least 3 weeks between eyebrow threading appointments, but as of late, a week after threading the hairs are already growing back!

11
CHOP CHOP – CUT BIT BY BIT

So you have your hair growth tips down, you've cut out all the crap and know what styles can get you through the hard times. Now what happens when your hair grows to a point where you have enough 'regrowth' compared to the damaged hair left over?

It is time my friend to pick up the scissors (or have someone else do it for you!).

Having my dry curly cut took my hairs health and look to a whole new level! 'Glow up' as they say! A good cut makes a great difference and I would only recommend cutting your hair whilst it's in its natural curly state instead of whilst straight because you will hardly wear your hair straight.

My past cuts have always been done on wet or straight hair, which doesn't look right when your hair is then curly. You want volume and shape with your curly cut.

Below are some keywords you can mention to potential stylists to see if they are experienced in certain techniques.

KEY WORDS

Dry cut, Curl by curl cut, Deva-cut, Deva specialist, and Big chop.

Big Chop

If in the beginning stages you feel that transitioning just isn't for you and you don't mind having your hair really short then go for a big chop! It will save you time and you can start with your hair instantly all over again by cutting off all of your damaged hair.

Curly Hair Specialist Salons in the UK

This is probably the question I get asked the most as a blogger! So many of us have lost trust in hairdressers and salons which I totally can relate too. We are so lucky that now the natural hair movement is so massive, and more and more stylists seem to be waking up!

Below are some curly hair salons/stylists that I have been too myself or have heard great reviews from.

3Thirty Salon – Based in East London this salon has beautiful décor and the owner Tiff is so friendly, she has years of experience dealing with curly hair, and I have heard great things about her curly hair styling. (Great for colouring and a cut).

Unruly Curls – An artsy looking salon with character! Ask for Michael Price the curl specialist.

Lindsey Hughes 'The Curl Whisperer' - My wonderful stylist! Lindsey first cut my hair in 2015 and I LOVED my results, it made my hair so much healthier, and it grew faster!

I am not sure about curly specialists in other parts of the UK but always ask for someone who is deva trained, or has knowledge of a dry cut or curl by curl cut.

With social media, nowadays you can instantly find a stylist and their speciality, so do some research beforehand.

Curly Hair Specialist Salons in the USA

You curlies are lucky! You pretty much have deva curl specialists in every state so I am sure finding a stylist won't be hard for you, again you can always do a search on Instagram for stylists and speak with your curl icons and find out where they get their hair styled.

Curly Hair Specialist Salons Internationally

Again use your social media and seach skills to find somewhere in your area.

DIY

I have never tried cutting my curls myself but there are 100's of tutorials on YouTube where curlies have successfully trimmed their own hair and made it look very easy. If DIY is your only option, give it a try carefully!

12
MAINTAIN THE MANE

By now you should have great confidence in starting your journey or have even been transitioning with the above tips for a while now. If all is going well that's great!! BUT this is also a lifetime commitment so below are my top tips for maintaining your hairs health and these are things I still do.

Satin Accessories

One of the 'major keys' of healthy hair care is to look after your curls whilst you sleep. I believe that this is really important and why I created my own satin hair accessories! I switched to satin scarfs and pillowcases at night time after watching tutorials online, and after the first few trials I noticed the difference straight away! I didn't know that it was possible to still wake up with defined curls! I was used to a fluff ball of knots in the morning.

Putting my hair up in a pineapple, with my satin scrunchies, (when it is defined and moisturised)

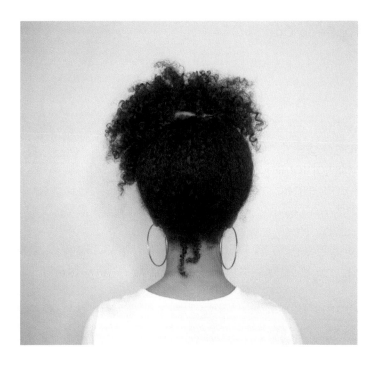

Tying with a satin scarf and then sleeping on my satin pillowcase keeps my hair moisturised, untangled and in place for the next day. This is because satin simply slips and is soft on your hair and skin whereas, cotton is rough, so you will get tangles and dry hair. Often you will find if you sleep on a cotton pillowcase there are hairs on your pillow in the morning, this is due to the friction and your hair getting caught in the cotton fibres.

Shop here www. osocurly. com

Heat For Deep Conditioning

This is a life changing hair tip right here! Especially for those with low porosity hair! Deep conditioning weekly alone is something you NEED to be doing as it penetrates the hair deeper than co-washing or your daily moisturiser. This gives your hair a great start to a new week. I always find that my hair feels lighter and softer after my deep conditioning treatments especially when applying a heated cap on top. If you haven't invested in a heated cap yet, you can still use heat by applying 2 shower caps in a steamy bathroom, wrapping a warm towel around your shower cap or sitting under a hooded dryer to warm up your treatment.

Shop here: https : // www. etsy. com /shop/ThermalHairCare/

Wide Tooth Combs & Brushes

To prevent unnecessary breakage you must be careful with the way you detangle your hair! Instead of tugging at your hair with any kind of brush or comb. You will need a wide tooth comb as it caters to the separation of the hair, and preserves your curls. If you prefer to use brushes I recommend the Denman brush as it is so easy to smooth through your hair, and it also gives great results, is that if you like your curls clumped together.

The Gram (Instagram)

I have to give a huge thanks to all of the naturals and natural hair pages on Instagram! Visualisation is a great way to get what you want from life and I feel the constant curl love every time I open the app, thanks to the pages I follow!

When these images are reinforced daily it will become so easy to want to continue your healthy hair journey, as you feel that you are not alone! Just don't get curl envy as that isn't healthy, love your hair, and love your curl pattern!

A few of my favourite pages to follow are:

@GoCurls

@UnconditionedRoots

@Healthy_Hair_Journey

@TeamNatural_

SIGNS YOU ARE DOING WELL

Throughout your journey you will pay attention to every little change you see in your hair and there are a few ways to gage how well your hair is progressing.

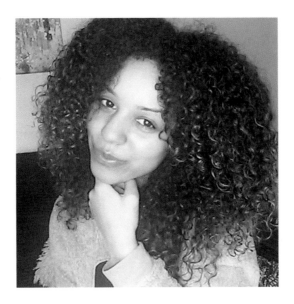

Transitioning (2015)

ELASTICITY

Your hair will actually stretch and return back to its shrunken curly state! This was something that my hair couldn't do for a very long time! Now I have shrinkage and know that it's a sign of health as my hair is moisturised and has elasticity.

STAYS MOISTURISED FOR LONGER

When you notice your hair can hold on to moisture for longer you will know that you are on the right track, this also comes down to the change in products you are using. A good leave-in conditioner should not make your hair feel and appear dry once your hair has dried from wash day.

NOTICABLE GROWTH

The most obvious sign of health is notable hair growth. For the journey you should do a length check every few months to monitor it's growth. During my time of constant hair damage my hair would not grow past my shoulders but now my hair grows way past my shoulders every 6 months or so after a cut!

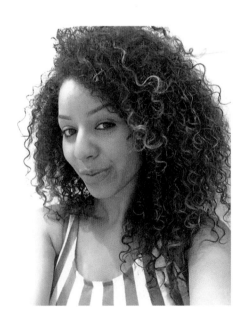

ENDS

You will notice that your hair curls all the way down from your root to your ends! No more split or dry ends should occur if you have grown out all of the damage and are maintaining your hair well.

13
SUCCESS STORIES

Below are 4 stories from girls that have followed my journey and started their own! I hope this will give you an extra push as it not only works for me but below is proof that transitioning to natural curls can work for you too!

MICA - London, UK

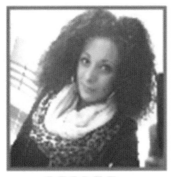

BEFORE

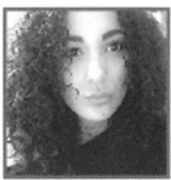

AFTER

How did you damage your hair?

It all started in year 7 or 8 when a lot of my friends were straightening their hair, I felt as like I was the only one whose mum was still doing their hair. My mum always had my hair in either cornrows, single plaits or bunches. I begged my mum for straighteners for a good year or so then she finally gave in and told me I'll learn the hard way if I don't look after my hair properly and surely I did!

The older I got the more I used them and started to lose care of my hair, I thought nothing would go wrong because it was long and thick. Once I hit college I got introduced to extensions and hair dye that was it I wanted long straight hair! I dyed my hair a lot and used all extension going from bonding glue to clip-ins and sew-ins. I would sometimes have my hair out 'curly' but it didn't look how it used to so I would just end up straightening it anyways.

I got fed up with straightening my hair all the time so I decided to relax my hair to make life easier but stupidly I dyed my hair a week after relaxing it and it was that day my hair just broke out. The texture, the length everything was gone, it was just horrible! That's when I knew it was time to stop or I would end up with hair I couldn't save.

Best advice/trick you learnt from UKCurlyGirl?

Once I stopped damaging my hair a friend of mine told me about Shannon and showed me her Instagram page and told me she would help me a lot. I went through her page and knew that she would definitely help me out! Shannon showed me that there is a lot of hair products made for different mixed race hair types and different techniques to help your hair that I never knew about. I was using anything for black or white people's hair. I love a wash and go! Being a mum I'm always running around juggling everything from school run to work so a wash and go is my life. I now know what to use/do and what not to thanks to Shannon.

Was there a time when you wanted to give up with your hair journey (and why)?

I haven't wanted to give up my journey because I look at how my hair looks and feels now. I do miss my hair straight and wearing extensions but I'd never go back. Sometimes I do get fed up especially when my hair gets overly knotty or my curls don't look how I want, I just got to Shannon's page and remind myself that this is fully worth it.

How long did your journey take or is currently taking?

I started my journey about 2/3 years ago but within the last year or so I've been on the ball making sure I reach my hair goal. My hair hasn't looked or felt this good in years and I'm sooo happy and grateful for Shannon's help.

Typical hair routine?

I do a wash and go routine every few days but I mostly wet my hair down with a spray bottle to detangle and moisturize my hair.

CHLOE-JADE - London, UK

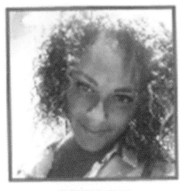

BEFORE

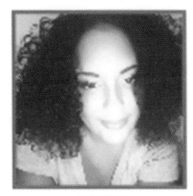

AFTER

How did you damage your hair?

I damaged my hair so much in the past that even talking about it stresses me. It started off at like 8 years old - some other mixed race girls I knew were getting their hair texturized and relaxed at the hairdressers - I guess their parents wanted an easy life.

It made me jealous and I was always begging my mum to let me try it. One day she gave in, with a do at home relaxer but weirdly it didn't take, my hair never lasted straight! I tried again when I was about 11 – it still didn't take so I gave up with the relaxer, and I started getting friends to straighten it for me like once every 6 months as they all had the GHD's that were the rage - but that didn't work for me either, the smallest amount of moisture and the ringlets sprung back into action! So I've never ever been a supporter of straightening techniques, as they never worked for me. I even tried a Brazilian blow dry a few years back - the most amount of rubbish I have ever wasted my money on!

I'm sure all that I've mentioned caused damage. At about 13 I started going on a mad one with hair dyes, reds, then blondes, then browns, alternatively. To top it off my go-to product in the younger years was the 30p gel that you used to buy from corner shops and pound shops etc. I then went on to use Palmers cocoa butter (for skin) in my hair for year's right up until about 2 years ago. I can't remember what sparked this I think I just tried it one day and stuck to it - so it's funny for me that now Palmers have a hair care range!

This continued right up until I was 24 and climaxed and begging my dad to BLEACH my hair in my kitchen with some hard-core bleach mix. He was very anti but I guess he thought he was helping me instead of me doing it myself. I was trying to reverse some colour so I could go from red to blonde. It went bright orange – literally, and I was devastated. I wasn't in a financial position to ever go to the hairdressers as I had young twins and so for 3 days I used a hat and scarf (in the summer) to go to the supermarket, nursery etc. until a friend bailed me out and sent me to the hairdressers.

I just went to the nearest one which was mainly an Asian place but they were shocked and I knew they had no experience of my hair. But an Arab lady sorted the colour out as best she could and it took hours, however the damage was bad it was dry, there was no curl left and people were asking me what I'd done to my hair, it wasn't straight nor curly it was just limp and lifeless, I was convinced at the time that it was irreversible - so when I began following Shannon it really gave me hope!

Best advice/trick you learnt from UKCurlyGirl?

The best thing was all the different products and using NATURAL hair products. Before seeing Shannon online I would use stuff for Caucasian hair that stank of alcohol and chemicals, and did nothing for my hair at all. The ingredients I dread to even think of now. So introducing me to a whole other world of healthy and natural hair products was the best tip and I haven't looked back since.

Learning about natural hair products and ways to keep curly hair textures healthy and nourished has been a saving grace because I have 6 year old twin girls one with hair just like mine and one with thicker and more afro hair. I now use only natural hair products in their hair and will apply a lot of UK Curly Girl's techniques whilst raising these girls and teaching them how to love and look after their hair.

Their journey will be a far cry from mine growing up so really a huge thanks Shannon I'm so glad I discovered you. My girls are now aware of what natural hair means and when they see ladies when we are out with big curly hair they say "look mummy its natural hair". It wasn't that long ago that they were begging for straight blonde hair and getting upset that they weren't like the majority at school. This journey has taught me things but also taught me to teach them and that is a really valuable lesson. Also another great tip I've had from Shannon is the regular deep treatments and protein treatments. I've realised they are essential.

Was there a time when you wanted to give up with your hair journey (and why)?

I've not wanted to give up as such - because I will never go back to those bad hair products - or to bleaching my hair etc. The only one thing that gets me through is knowing my hair has the ability to be similar to Shannon's (as from following you and seeing the before and after pictures) I've noticed we have a similar hair type. But it just doesn't grow or thrive how I want it to (although I do keep cutting the split ends) and the volume that I want just isn't happening.

I do often wonder where I'm going wrong, but when I feel like that I do realise there is a difference in my hairs health and funnily enough I look at pictures of Shannon particularly the before ones that remind me so much of my old hair when it was at its worst and it gives me hope when I see how far she has come!

How long did your journey take or is currently taking?

I have been on this journey for about 8 months now - and it is definitely still ongoing. I hope and pray for the day when my hair looks as great and thick as Shannon's and others that I follow! I'm really excited to continue to try and get the best results and healthiest hair possible - I do have hope. I've got so many products and brands.

A drawer full of things so hopefully soon, I will find my go to miracle product and get into a really good routine.

Typical hair routine and products that have worked for you?

I put product on and do a simple flat twist/bun style most days until a few days after the wash when the hair is bouncy enough for me to start wearing it out for a few days before wash again. It's not the best routine - I am dying to master a wash and go but first I need that volume and growth before I have the confidence. I do find a lot of products quite heavy though so I am still learning, and trying to find a few miracle products that my hair loves and that work perfectly for me. Fingers crossed!

BROOKE – Stockport, UK

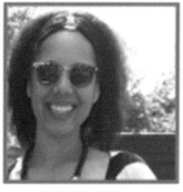

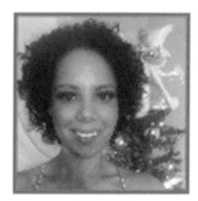

BEFORE **AFTER**

How did you damage your hair?

My hair was damaged through chemical relaxing for about 18 years. Until I was 10/11 years old I had thick bushy hair, the curls were never really defined mainly because my mum didn't know how to manage them and I remember a lot of tears before school because she was brushing through my dry hair, it would then be put into pigtails or a pony.

At that age I never really thought about the difference in my hair compared to the other girls in a predominately white school. But by the time I joined high school I noticed the difference and would be jealous at how easily the other girls could wash and comb their hair and the versatility it had. This is when I began relaxing my hair. My first experience wasn't a particularly good one. My hairdresser asked me to let her know if I felt any tingling whilst the chemical relaxer was on, after about ten minutes

I felt burning but didn't say anything scared that the relaxer wouldn't take. So as a result when it was eventually washed off I was left with a burnt scalp, which hurt to brush for weeks after. Admittedly the results were exactly what I wanted at the time and I fitted in with my peers.

Best advice/tricks you've learnt from UK Curly Girl?

The best advice I've learnt from UK Curly Girl is to have patience and that it is ok to have setbacks, such as a bit of heat or colour damage, it's all part of the journey.

Practically, UKCurlyGirl has given me good advice on how to tame frizz and how to master a wash n go – wash with warm, rinse with cold, use a cotton t-shirt to dry, use a leave in and brush with a Denman brush. None of which I would've done without watching the You Tube videos.

Was there a time when you wanted to give up (and why)?

I've wanted to give up frequently, not to go back to the chemical relaxer but to blow dry and use straighteners daily. The urge to do this has been strong when going on dates and I've felt very unconfident with my "new" hair, because I didn't really know what to do with it and I would be nervous as to what guys would think of it.

How long did your journey take or is taking?

My journey back to natural started in 2012 after I went to the hairdressers and asked them to make my hair curly, the hairdresser explained that it was literally impossible because the relaxer had permanently straightened my hair and that the only thing I could do was to grow it out. Weirdly, that was the first time it occurred to me that I'd damaged my hair beyond repair, which was a massive wakeup call and quote upsetting.

At first I blow dried my hair once or twice a week and had regular trims. Then after following people like UKCurlyGirl on Instagram I learnt how to look after my hair properly whilst transitioning and stopped the blow- dries completely in November 2015. At this point my hair was past my shoulders, but still had a lot of heat damage, so I took the plunge, found a curly hairdresser and asked them to cut it all off. My first reaction was to cry as my hair was up to my ears but 4 months on, it's growing rapidly and is in the best condition it's been in for years (minus a little bit of heat damage at the front).

Typical hair routine?

I wash and deep condition my hair once a week and wrap my hair in cling film and leave for approx. 30 minutes. I rinse out and apply Tresseme natural's conditioner (all over) and Organix Kukui de-frizz conditioner (on the top of my head), detangle and rinse out using cold water. I then apply Shea Moisture Black Jamaican castor oil leave in conditioner brush through with a Denman and apply vegetable glycerine oil (my hair loves this stuff). Once a month I will also use the ApHogee 2 minute Keratin reconstructor.

AZZA – Plymouth, UK

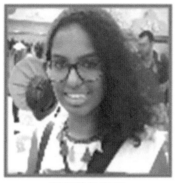 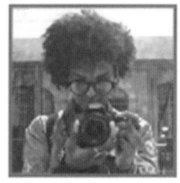

BEFORE **AFTER**

How did you damage your hair?

When I was 15/16 years old, I used to constantly straighten my hair for school. I felt that straightening my hair would make me feel better about myself and make me fit in with everyone else in my year. At that time, I didn't realise how much damage I was doing to my hair, until I spoke to my cousins and their hair was so long and curly and it made me think; "How did they get their hair like that?" I would constantly ask them for tips on how to make it better and healthier.

Through trial and error, I got to a stage where I realised how dead the ends of my hair was and I took it upon myself to get a professional haircut. I got my hair cut in the Priory Bellshill in Glasgow, while I was staying with my best friend. The woman who cut my hair, talked to me for hours about how my hair needed a cut desperately and what I can do to make it better after the cut.

After the haircut, I saw how healthy my hair was and I know I didn't want to go back to the way it was before, so I talked to my cousins again and they helped me pick the best products for my hair type and just keep experimenting until I find the right combination. Having my hair natural, has made me see myself in a different light; stronger more confident and that I can embrace it more. This is something I have always wanted to feel in life.

Best advice/trick you learnt from UKCurlyGirl?

The best advice that I have learnt is to go through hours of research and watch videos about curly hair/natural hair journey. This defiantly helped me and inspired me to stay on my journey.

Was there a time when you wanted to give up with your hair journey (and why)?

I wanted to give up on my hair when I was in University in Dubai. I knew how badly damaged it was from when I left the UK, and seeing my cousins look after their hair and the results that they had, made me realise I need to start looking after my hair.

How long did your journey take or is currently taking?

My journey started on and off in 2013 and the summer of 2014. But I started looking after my hair properly, last year and completely stop using hair products and heat damage tools, unless I really need to. Since I made that decision, I have been getting so much love and support from friends and family and now I feel more confident.

Typical hair routine and products that have worked for you?

My hair routine would be on the 5th day, when my hair would be at a "dread loc" stage, so I would cleanse it with my shampoo (a very small palm sized) two times. Just to make sure it was 100% clean, then I would condition my hair and leave it in for 10/15mins and rinse 70% of it out and leave the rest in. Then afterwards, I would use my curly hair gels and creams to maintain the curls. I am currently using a combination of OGX Shampoo and Conditioner and Deva-Curl No Poo Shampoo and Conditioner, to wash my hair with. For styling, I have been using a mix of Lush's R&B Cream, Shea Moisture Coconut and Hibiscus Curl Enhancer and Eco Styler Argan Oil Gel. If I feel my hair needs more moisture, I will make a hair mask with Avocado, Olive Oil, Banana and Mayonnaise.

14
EXPERT ADVICE

So you have heard from me, some of my followers and if you still aren't convinced have a read of what some hair care 'experts' have to say on the topic of transitioning!

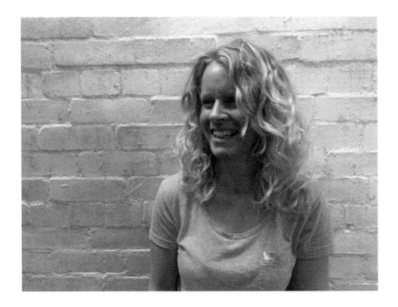

Lindsey 'Curl Whisperer' – Curly Hair Stylist

"Don't give up! Keep practicing and seek advice from a curly professional who can start you off on the right setting rather than listening to other curlies with different hair types."

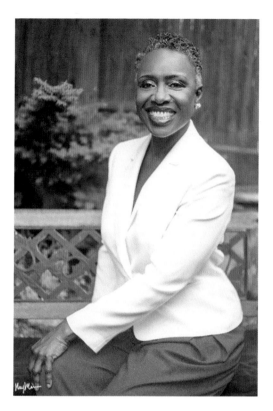

Diane C. Bailey – Celebrity Stylist & SheaMoisture Brand Ambassador

"Transitioning hair is very fragile, because there are two textures on one strand. It's vital to strengthen the shaft where the two textures meet with ingredients that are rich in fatty acids and vitamins, such as Jamaican black castor oil. I recommend SheaMoisture, Jamaican Black Castor Oil Strengthen & Restore Masque to aid in fortifying the follicle, and detangling hair to discourage breakage and splits ends. Apply the masque, then cover hair with a plastic cap and add soothing steam to open the cuticle for intense moisture.

For styling during transitioning, wear your hair in protective styles to reduce hair manipulation and breakage, such as rod sets, cornrow sets, twists sets, braids or twists with/without extensions. When transitioning, select styles that allow you to wear your hair freely without added stress from tight extensions. However, if you do decide to rock your extensions, make sure you keep your hair moisturized to avoid it from becoming brittle and breaking."

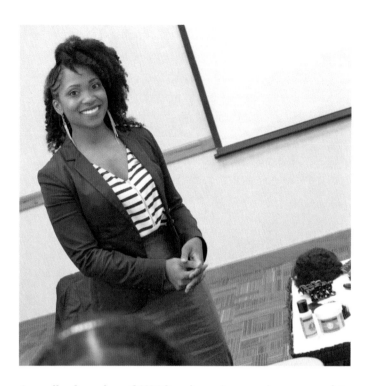

Janelle Sands – CURLS educator and owner of Secret Curl Society

"The battle ahead is both physical and emotional. It will require maturity and commitment! On the physical side, there will be a degree of "let go" that is necessary to move forward. Therefore at the onset of the journey, I advise Transitioners to commit to trimming their hair once every other month on a regular basis until they are emotionally and physically ready for the big chop. To delay the scissors for 1 year or more can be detrimental and will definitely make the big chop harder to accomplish without deep heartbreak.

Emotionally, I would remind transitioners that they are not becoming a new version of themselves, but rather a "purer" version of themselves which may require more work in some areas and less work in other areas. Nevertheless, it'll be GREAT!!!! Congrats in advance!!!"

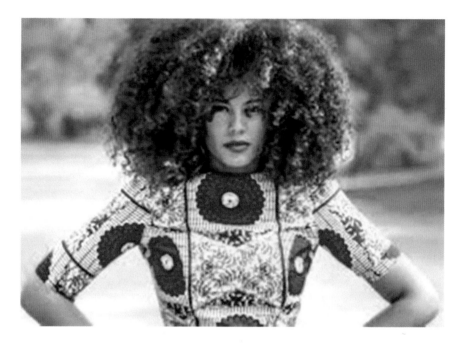

Simone Powderley (@HairIsSimba Hair Model/Brand Influencer)

"SAY NO TO HEAT! Pack it all up! Then you begin with treatments, once a week give your hair the loving it deserves. Deep conditioner, Mask or oil treatment! Admire other naturals but remember your journey is journey! Embrace every part of it and take plenty of selfies, here is to healthy hair!"

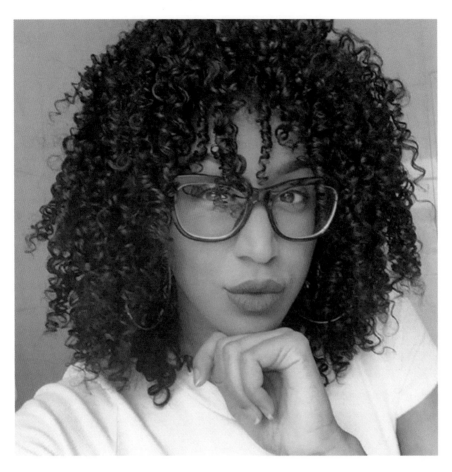

Helana Richardson (@Helzzzrich Hair/Food Blogger)

"Be consistent and patient, it usually looks worse before it looks better! Deep condition regularly, cut the damaged & dead ends off and just embrace your nature state!"

15
FINALE

So there you have it! Everything you will need to start your transitioning hair journey. I hope this book has inspired you to stop damaging your hair, and learn to love you, and what grows naturally from your scalp! So many of us have grown up believing our hair is in the 'other' category, isn't normal, and isn't attractive, but I am here to tell you that this is FALSE! Curly girls are out here winning!

Good luck on your journeys, and I hope to see all of your amazing results as I believe you can do it!

Thanks to the following:

This book has been in the making for the past year but has really been in the making since I was a young child. Writing has always been something I was good at. One of my very first memories from school was a parents evening where my English teacher told my mum "Shannon will be a writer one day" and it's crazy how I never really wanted to be one, but everything comes full circle.

So many thanks to Mr Chapman for seeing the talent I had back then! I also want to thank vlogger SunKissAlba for inspiring me to start transitioning, she gave me the confidence and knowledge I desperately needed!

I also want to thank my favourite brand Shea Moisture for creating products that actually MOISTURISE my hair and giving me hope in my naturalness.

Huge thanks to my loved ones who pushed me to get this done! And to the Internet and 1000's of curly girls online that inspire me every single day!

And last but definitely not least, YOU I thank YOU for even reading this book, following me on social media, watching my tutorials. Every single comment you leave means a lot to me and keeps me going. There is no better feeling than knowing you are inspiring others in a positive way.

Let's keep going curlies!

Until next time keep embracing your naturalness!

Make sure you follow me on all social accounts @ukcurlygirl and subscribe to my mail list via ukcurlygirl.com to keep up to date with my latest posts.

32644695R00077

Printed in Poland
by Amazon Fulfillment
Poland Sp. z o.o., Wrocław